iCare
Extra Forms

Photozig, Inc.

iCare Extra Forms:

iCare® Extra Forms is part of an informative program developed by Photozig, Inc. in collaboration with Stanford University, Alzheimer's Association, and other organizations, which was funded by the National Institute on Aging (part of the National Institutes of Health), and specifically created for caregivers of individuals with dementia or memory loss.

The educational iCare program describes the skills on how to cope with caregiving, reduce related distress, and improve the quality of life of caregivers and loved ones.

For additional information, please go to the iCare web site at: **www.icarefamily.com**

Contact Us:

Any questions about the iCare project should be addressed to the project staff at Photozig, Inc:

icare@photozig.com

www.icarefamily.com

Important Notes:

The instructions and advice presented here are in no way intended as a substitute for professional medical judgment and assistance. It is not intended to treat any medical or psychological problems. This publication is an educational tool only, to help you learn more about dementia and to give you information about common ways to cope with related problems. Not all of the information provided is suitable for everyone, and we do not guarantee or promise that the techniques illustrated in this publication will be helpful to every individual caregiver who watches related DVD or reads/uses this publication. For example, the problems you are confronted with may be different from the ones presented here, or you may have so many problems that you are overwhelmed and in need of professional assistance in order to cope effectively with your situation. Individuals with medical conditions should not use the "Deep Breathing" or any of the techniques presented here for stress management without their doctor's advice and approval. To reduce the risk of injury, consult your doctor before beginning this or any caregiver program. The instructions and advice presented here are in no way intended as a substitute for family counseling, psychotherapy, or any form of medical treatment.

Acknowledgments:

This project is supported by Award Number R44AG032762 from the National Institute on Aging. The content is solely the responsibility of the authors and does not necessarily represent the official views of the National Institute on Aging or the National Institutes of Health.

Credits

Research Team

Bruno Kajiyama, MS
Principal Investigator, Photozig, Inc.

Dolores Gallagher-Thompson, PhD, ABPP
Co-Principal Investigator
Stanford University School of Medicine

Larry Thompson, PhD
Co-Principal Investigator
Stanford University School of Medicine

Photozig Healthcare Research
Irene Rivera-Valverde, BA, MFTT
John Di Mario, BS
Marian Tzuang, MSW
Mio Yamashita, MA, ATR, MFT
Tamiko Eto-Iwase, MA

Advisory Committee

David Coon, PhD
Arizona State University

Elizabeth Edgerly, PhD
Alzheimer's Association of Northern California & Northern Nevada

Ladson Hinton, MD
UC Davis Medical School & UC Davis Alzheimer's Disease Center

Suzann Ogland-Hand, PhD
Pine Rest Christian Mental Health Service

For further information, please visit **www.icarefamily.com**

We would like to thank all organizations that supported this project, including the National Institutes of Health (NIH), Alzheimer's Association, NASA, and Stanford University.

This research was substantially supported by grant R44AG032762 from NIH, entitled "iCare Stress Management e-Training for Dementia Family Caregivers," to Bruno Kajiyama.

Table of Contents:

iCare Extra Forms: Background Information

The publication contains extra copies of the forms from the *iCare Handbook*, which was created to work hand-in-hand with the iCare video training for caregivers of older adults with Alzheimer's or dementia. If you need quick instructions for the forms, you can also check the *iCare Handbook Express*, which gives you quick access to the most frequently used forms from the video training program.

This is not intended to replace the complete *iCare Handbook*. Please see the *iCare Handbook* for detailed explanations and background information, including examples, resources, and a glossary of helpful words.

For more information, please visit: **www.icarefamily.com**

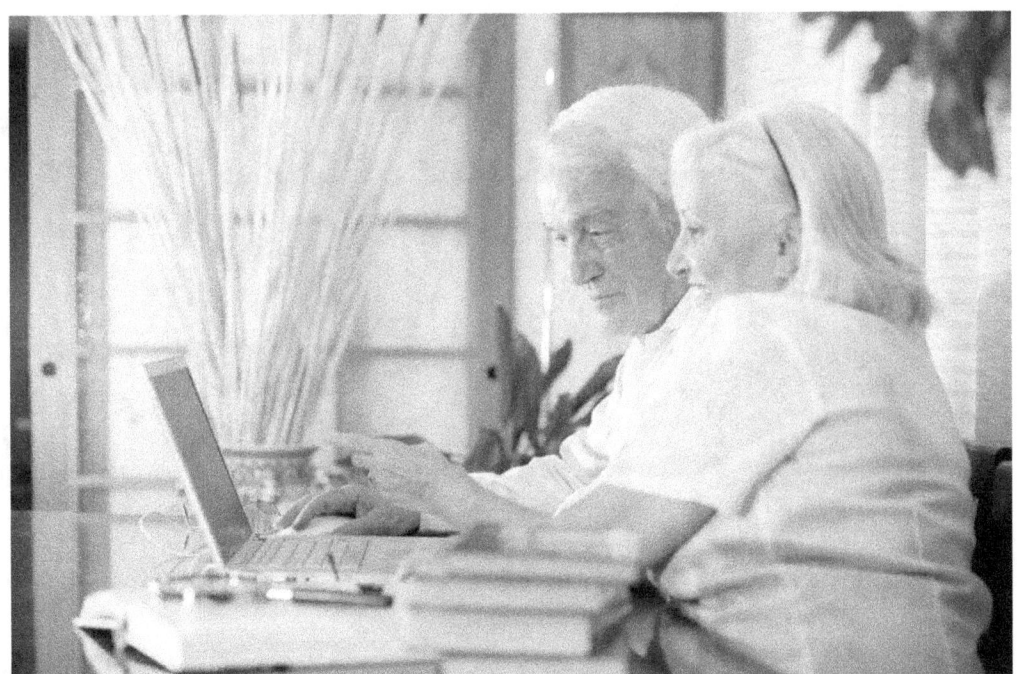

My Action Plan

Review *(what did I learn in this chapter?)*

Goal *(what do I want to accomplish?)*

Problems *(what might get in the way?)* | **Solutions** *(how to work around problems)*

I can do it *(rate your confidence level)*

Definitely Not					Maybe				Definitely Yes
1	2	3	4	5	6	7	8	9	10

Actions *(what needs to be done, how, when, where, etc.)*

- -

Save this for follow up later (aim for within one to two weeks)

Notes *(What worked? What did not work? How can it be improved?)*

The more you practice the skills, the more likely you are to feel better about yourself ☺

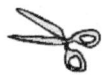

My Action Plan

Review *(what did I learn in this chapter?)*

Goal *(what do I want to accomplish?)*

Problems *(what might get in the way?)* | **Solutions** *(how to work around problems)*

I can do it *(rate your confidence level)*

Definitely Not   **Maybe**   **Definitely Yes**

1	2	3	4	5	6	7	8	9	10

Actions *(what needs to be done, how, when, where, etc.)*

Save this for follow up later (aim for within one to two weeks)

Notes *(What worked? What did not work? How can it be improved?)*

The more you practice the skills, the more likely you are to feel better about yourself ☺

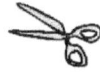

My Action Plan

Review *(what did I learn in this chapter?)*

Goal *(what do I want to accomplish?)*

Problems *(what might get in the way?)*

Solutions *(how to work around problems)*

I can do it *(rate your confidence level)*

Definitely Not					Maybe				Definitely Yes
1	2	3	4	5	6	7	8	9	10

Actions *(what needs to be done, how, when, where, etc.)*

Save this for follow up later *(aim for within one to two weeks)*

Notes *(What worked? What did not work? How can it be improved?)*

The more you practice the skills, the more likely you are to feel better about yourself ☺

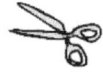

My Action Plan

Review *(what did I learn in this chapter?)*

Goal *(what do I want to accomplish?)*

Problems *(what might get in the way?)* | **Solutions** *(how to work around problems)*

I can do it *(rate your confidence level)*

Definitely Not					Maybe				Definitely Yes
1	2	3	4	5	6	7	8	9	10

Actions *(what needs to be done, how, when, where, etc.)*

Save this for follow up later (aim for within one to two weeks)

Notes *(What worked? What did not work? How can it be improved?)*

The more you practice the skills, the more likely you are to feel better about yourself ☺

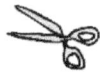

My Action Plan

Review *(what did I learn in this chapter?)*

Goal *(what do I want to accomplish?)*

Problems *(what might get in the way?)*

Solutions *(how to work around problems)*

I can do it *(rate your confidence level)*

Definitely Not					Maybe				Definitely Yes
1	2	3	4	5	6	7	8	9	10

Actions *(what needs to be done, how, when, where, etc.)*

- -

Save this for follow up later (aim for within one to two weeks)

Notes *(What worked? What did not work? How can it be improved?)*

The more you practice the skills, the more likely you are to feel better about yourself ☺

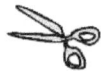

My Action Plan

Review *(what did I learn in this chapter?)*

Goal *(what do I want to accomplish?)*

Problems *(what might get in the way?)*	Solutions *(how to work around problems)*

I can do it *(rate your confidence level)*

Definitely Not					Maybe				Definitely Yes
1	2	3	4	5	6	7	8	9	10

Actions *(what needs to be done, how, when, where, etc.)*

- -

Save this for follow up later (aim for within one to two weeks)

Notes *(What worked? What did not work? How can it be improved?)*

The more you practice the skills, the more likely you are to feel better about yourself ☺

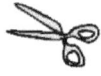

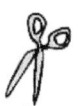

My Thought Record

Situation:

1. Current Thoughts	2. Feelings	3. Challenge the Thought	4. Replacement *What is a more creative or assertive way of thinking?*	5. Future Actions *How will I react differently next time?*

My Thought Record

Situation:

1. Current Thoughts	2. Feelings	3. Challenge the Thought	4. Replacement *What is a more creative or assertive way of thinking?*	5. Future Actions *How will I react differently next time?*

17

18

My Thought Record

Situation:

1. Current Thoughts	2. Feelings	3. Challenge the Thought	4. Replacement *What is a more creative or assertive way of thinking?*	5. Future Actions *How will I react differently next time?*

19

Pleasant Activities Log

- List **<u>Pleasant Activities</u>** that you plan to do this week.
- Place a check mark next to each activity that you tried.
- Count how many activities you did each day.

Pleasant Activities	Mon /__	Tue /	Wed /	Thu /	Fri /	Sat /	Sun /
1.							
2.							
3.							
4.							
5.							
6.							
7.							
8							
9.							
10.							
Totals for each day:							

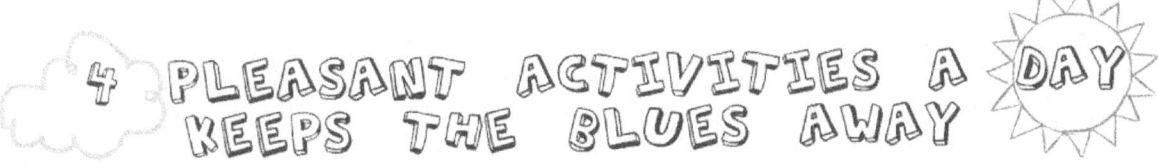

4 PLEASANT ACTIVITIES A DAY
KEEPS THE BLUES AWAY

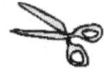

Pleasant Activities Log

- List **<u>Pleasant Activities</u>** that you plan to do this week.
- Place a check mark next to each activity that you tried.
- Count how many activities you did each day.

Pleasant Activities	Mon _/_	Tue _/_	Wed _/_	Thu _/_	Fri _/_	Sat _/_	Sun _/_
1.							
2.							
3.							
4.							
5.							
6.							
7.							
8							
9.							
10.							
Totals for each day:							

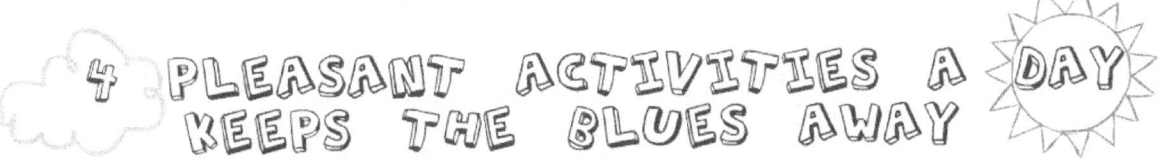

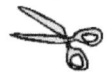

Pleasant Activities Log

- List **Pleasant Activities** that you plan to do this week.
- Place a check mark next to each activity that you tried.
- Count how many activities you did each day.

Pleasant Activities	Mon _/_	Tue _/_	Wed _/_	Thu _/_	Fri _/_	Sat _/_	Sun _/_
1.							
2.							
3.							
4.							
5.							
6.							
7.							
8							
9.							
10.							
Totals for each day:							

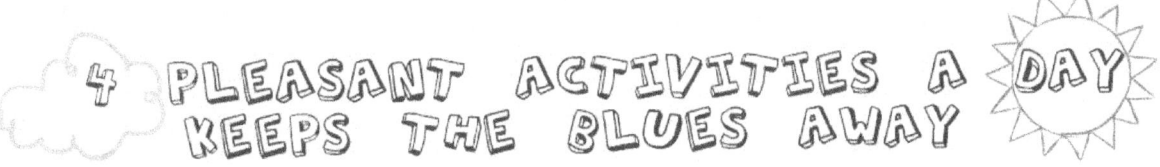

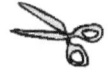

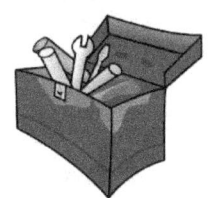
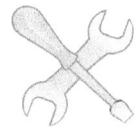

The "Nuts and Bolts" of Pleasant Activities

As we mentioned during the Pleasant Activities Plan, the idea is to commit to doing something for yourself on a regular basis. An excellent way to plan anything is to write out what you plan on doing and how you plan to do it. To help you in planning out your activity, we have provided a Nuts and Bolts of Pleasant Activities worksheet below. Please use this for each activity you try out. This will help avoid disappointing results due to forgetting to bring something or not remembering a necessary part of that activity.

Happy Event:	
Where?	
When? (when, how often, how long)	
What's needed? (materials, things to bring)	
How? (arrangements and steps)	

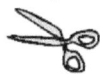

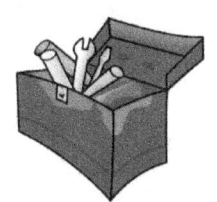

The "Nuts and Bolts" of Pleasant Activities

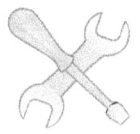

As we mentioned during the Pleasant Activities Plan, the idea is to commit to doing something for yourself on a regular basis. An excellent way to plan anything is to write out what you plan on doing and how you plan to do it. To help you in planning out your activity, we have provided a Nuts and Bolts of Pleasant Activities worksheet below. Please use this for each activity you try out. This will help avoid disappointing results due to forgetting to bring something or not remembering a necessary part of that activity.

Happy Event:	
Where?	
When? (*when, how often, how long*)	
What's needed? (*materials, things to bring*)	
How? (*arrangements and steps*)	

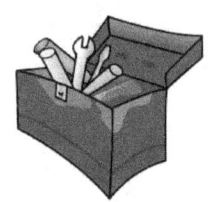

The "Nuts and Bolts" of Pleasant Activities

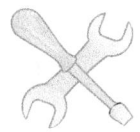

As we mentioned during the Pleasant Activities Plan, the idea is to commit to doing something for yourself on a regular basis. An excellent way to plan anything is to write out what you plan on doing and how you plan to do it. To help you in planning out your activity, we have provided a Nuts and Bolts of Pleasant Activities worksheet below. Please use this for each activity you try out. This will help avoid disappointing results due to forgetting to bring something or not remembering a necessary part of that activity.

Happy Event:	
Where?	
When? **(when, how often, how long)**	
What's needed? **(materials, things to bring)**	
How? **(arrangements and steps)**	

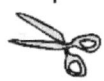

The "Nuts and Bolts" of Pleasant Activities
(For My Loved One and Me)

Pleasant activities can make the best use of a person's remaining abilities and can also reduce problematic behavior like wandering or agitation.

Because we want you to be successful in planning pleasant activities for both you and your loved one, we have put together a list of questions you should ask yourself beforehand so that things will go as smoothly as possible.

Think about the activity you have selected to enjoy with your loved one this week, and use the worksheet below to plan out your activity.

Happy Event:	
Where?	
When? (*when, how often, how long*)	
What's needed? (*materials, things to bring*)	
How? (*arrangements and steps*)	

The "Nuts and Bolts" of Pleasant Activities
(For My Loved One and Me)

Pleasant activities can make the best use of a person's remaining abilities and can also reduce problematic behavior like wandering or agitation.

Because we want you to be successful in planning pleasant activities for both you and your loved one, we have put together a list of questions you should ask yourself beforehand so that things will go as smoothly as possible.

Think about the activity you have selected to enjoy with your loved one this week, and use the worksheet below to plan out your activity.

Happy Event:	
Where?	
When? *(when, how often, how long)*	
What's needed? *(materials, things to bring)*	
How? *(arrangements and steps)*	

The "Nuts and Bolts" of Pleasant Activities
(For My Loved One and Me)

Pleasant activities can make the best use of a person's remaining abilities and can also reduce problematic behavior like wandering or agitation.

Because we want you to be successful in planning pleasant activities for both you and your loved one, we have put together a list of questions you should ask yourself beforehand so that things will go as smoothly as possible.

Think about the activity you have selected to enjoy with your loved one this week, and use the worksheet below to plan out your activity.

Happy Event:	
Where?	
When? (*when, how often, how long*)	
What's needed? (*materials, things to bring*)	
How? (*arrangements and steps*)	

Pleasant Activities Log for
My Loved One and Me

- List **Pleasant Activities** that you plan to do with your loved one this week.
- Place a check mark next to each activity that you tried.
- Count how many activities you did each day.

Pleasant Activities	Mon __/__	Tue __/__	Wed __/__	Thu __/__	Fri __/__	Sat __/__	Sun __/__
1.							
2.							
3.							
4.							
5.							
6.							
7.							
8.							
9.							
10.							
Totals for each day:							

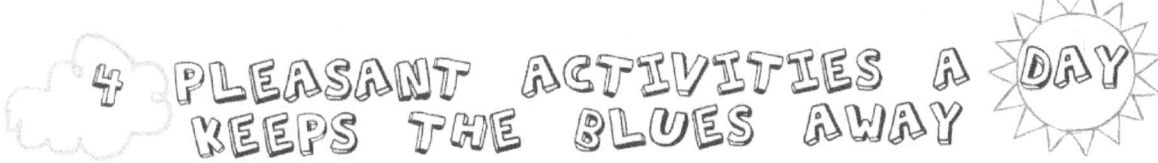

4 PLEASANT ACTIVITIES A DAY
KEEPS THE BLUES AWAY

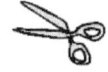

Pleasant Activities Log for
My Loved One and Me

- List **Pleasant Activities** that you plan to do with your loved one this week.
- Place a check mark next to each activity that you tried.
- Count how many activities you did each day.

Pleasant Activities	Mon _/_	Tue _/_	Wed _/_	Thu _/_	Fri _/_	Sat _/_	Sun _/_
1.							
2.							
3.							
4.							
5.							
6.							
7.							
8.							
9.							
10.							
Totals for each day:							

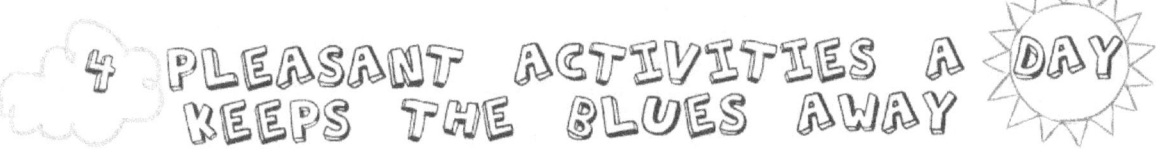

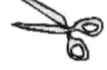

41

Pleasant Activities Log for
My Loved One and Me

- List **<u>Pleasant Activities</u>** that you plan to do with your loved one this week.
- Place a check mark next to each activity that you tried.
- Count how many activities you did each day.

Pleasant Activities	Mon _/_	Tue _/_	Wed _/_	Thu _/_	Fri _/_	Sat _/_	Sun _/_
1.							
2.							
3.							
4.							
5.							
6.							
7.							
8.							
9.							
10.							
Totals for each day:							

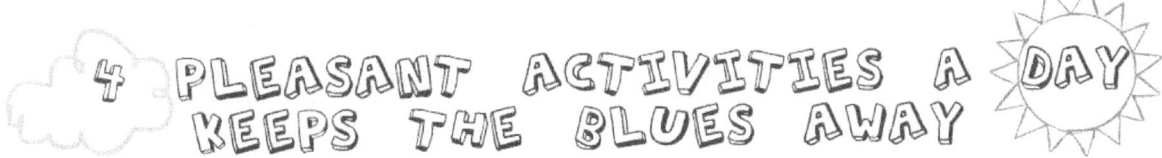

4 PLEASANT ACTIVITIES A DAY
KEEPS THE BLUES AWAY

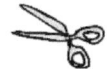

Communication Check Sheet

Take notes on how you communicated this week with your loved one—both verbally and nonverbally. **In Section A**: Explain what actually happened. In **Section B**: Write down: **(1)** what style of communication you used, **(2)** how it turned out and **(3)** how you felt about it afterwards.

Section A.

What I said or did to communicate with my loved one:

_____

_____

_____

_____

_____

_____

_____

Section B.

Style of Communication Used	How it Turned Out	How I Felt
_____	_____	_____
_____	_____	_____
_____	_____	_____
_____	_____	_____
_____	_____	_____
_____	_____	_____

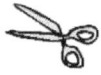

Communication Check Sheet

Take notes on how you communicated this week with your loved one—both verbally and nonverbally. **In Section A**: Explain what actually happened. In **Section B**: Write down: **(1)** what style of communication you used, **(2)** how it turned out and **(3)** how you felt about it afterwards.

Section A.

What I said or did to communicate with my loved one:

_____
_____
_____
_____
_____
_____

Section B.

Style of Communication Used	How it Turned Out	How I Felt
_____	_____	_____
_____	_____	_____
_____	_____	_____
_____	_____	_____
_____	_____	_____
_____	_____	_____

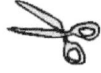

Communication Check Sheet

Take notes on how you communicated this week with your loved one—both verbally and nonverbally. **In Section A**: Explain what actually happened. In **Section B**: Write down: **(1)** what style of communication you used, **(2)** how it turned out and **(3)** how you felt about it afterwards.

Section A.

What I said or did to communicate with my loved one:

_____
_____
_____
_____
_____
_____
_____

Section B.

Style of Communication Used	How it Turned Out	How I Felt

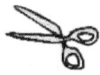

Medication List for Doctor's Appointment

Patient Name: _____

Drug Name	What It's for and Description of Pill (what it looks like)	Doctor	Dose	Instructions

Check with your primary doctor before stopping meds or taking any new medication from another doctor or a new over-the-counter drug.

Medication List for Doctor's Appointment

Patient Name: _____

Drug Name	What It's for and Description of Pill (what it looks like)	Doctor	Dose	Instructions

Check with your primary doctor before stopping meds or taking any new medication from another doctor or a new over-the-counter drug.

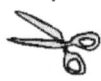

Medication List for Doctor's Appointment

Patient Name: _____

Drug Name	What It's for and Description of Pill (what it looks like)	Doctor	Dose	Instructions
Check with your primary doctor before stopping meds or taking any new medication from another doctor or a new over-the-counter drug.				

Medication List for Doctor's Appointment

Patient Name: _____

Drug Name	What It's for and Description of Pill (what it looks like)	Doctor	Dose	Instructions
Check with your primary doctor before stopping meds or taking any new medication from another doctor or a new over-the-counter drug.				

Medication List for Doctor's Appointment

Patient Name: _____

Drug Name	What It's for and Description of Pill (what it looks like)	Doctor	Dose	Instructions

Check with your primary doctor before stopping meds or taking any new medication from another doctor or a new over-the-counter drug.

Medication List for Doctor's Appointment

Patient Name: _____

Drug Name	What It's for and Description of Pill (what it looks like)	Doctor	Dose	Instructions

Check with your primary doctor before stopping meds or taking any new medication from another doctor or a new over-the-counter drug.

Doctor's Visit Worksheet

Concerns: _____
1. _____
2. _____
3. _____

_____

Notes: _____

_____
_____
_____
_____
_____
_____
_____

- ✂

Doctor's Visit Worksheet

Concerns: _____
1. _____
2. _____
3. _____

_____

Notes: _____

_____
_____
_____
_____
_____
_____
_____

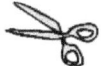

Doctor's Visit Worksheet

Concerns: _____

1. _____
2. _____
3. _____

_____

Notes: _____

_____
_____
_____
_____
_____
_____

- ✂

Doctor's Visit Worksheet

Concerns: _____

1. _____
2. _____
3. _____

Notes: _____

_____
_____
_____
_____
_____
_____

Doctor's Visit Worksheet

Concerns:
1.
2.
3.

Notes:

Doctor's Visit Worksheet

Concerns:
1.
2.
3.

Notes:

T-B-R RECORD SHEET

Use this form to record what has worked and not worked when you tried to figure out how to better manage your loved one's behaviors.

INSTRUCTIONS: **1.** Identify the problem behavior. **2.** Think about the trigger—what led up to the problem behavior? **3.** Recall how you reacted/responded to the problem behavior **4.** Think of a strategy to try that will EITHER change the trigger or your reaction to that problem. **5.** Lastly, observe what happened after you used this strategy, and fill in the last blank.

Date/ Day of Week	Time	Person(s) Present	Trigger ⟶ Behavior ⟶ Response		The Strategy I used to Change the Behavior
			2.	**1.** / **3.**	**4.**
					What Happened after you used this Strategy?
					5.

T-B-R RECORD SHEET

Use this form to record what has worked and not worked when you tried to figure out how to better manage your loved one's behaviors.

INSTRUCTIONS: **1.** Identify the problem behavior. **2.** Think about the trigger—what led up to the problem behavior? **3.** Recall how you reacted/responded to the problem behavior **4.** Think of a strategy to try that will EITHER change the trigger or your reaction to that problem. **5.** Lastly, observe what happened after you used this strategy, and fill in the last blank.

Date/ Day of Week	Time	Person(s) Present	Trigger ⟶ Behavior ⟶ Response		The Strategy I used to Change the Behavior
			2.	**1.**	**4.**
				3.	What Happened after you used this Strategy?
					5.

T-B-R RECORD SHEET

Use this form to record what has worked and not worked when you tried to figure out how to better manage your loved one's behaviors.

INSTRUCTIONS: **1.** Identify the problem behavior. **2.** Think about the trigger—what led up to the problem behavior. **3.** Recall how you reacted/responded to the problem behavior **4.** Think of a strategy to try that will EITHER change the trigger or your reaction to that problem. **5.** Lastly, observe what happened after you used this strategy, and fill in the last blank.

Date/ Day of Week	Time	Person(s) Present	Trigger ⟶	Behavior ⟶	Response	The Strategy I used to Change the Behavior
			2.	**1.**	**3.**	**4.**
						What Happened after you used this Strategy?
						5.

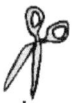

Healthy Habits Thought Record

(Thought Record for the Healthy Habits Chapter)

Situation:

Current thoughts	How do I feel about that?	What's keeping me from doing this differently?	Brainstorm: How can I make this work?	Goal for next time

69

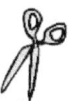

Healthy Habits Thought Record

(Thought Record for the Healthy Habits Chapter)

Situation:

Current thoughts	How do I feel about that?	What's keeping me from doing this differently?	Brainstorm: How can I make this work?	Goal for next time

71

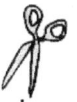

Healthy Habits Thought Record

(Thought Record for the Healthy Habits Chapter)

Situation:

Current thoughts	How do I feel about that?	What's keeping me from doing this differently?	Brainstorm: How can I make this work?	Goal for next time

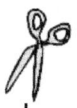

Chart to Help Me Plan Healthy Meals for the Week

Food for the Week

Dates: from _____ to _____

	Sunday	Monday	Tuesday	Wednesday	Thursday	Friday	Saturday
Morning							
Lunch							
Dinner							

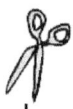

Chart to Help Me Plan Healthy Meals for the Week

Food for the Week
Dates: from _____ to _____

	Sunday	Monday	Tuesday	Wednesday	Thursday	Friday	Saturday
Morning							
Lunch							
Dinner							

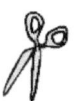

Chart to Help Me Plan Healthy Meals for the Week

Food for the Week

Dates: from _____ to _____

	Sunday	Monday	Tuesday	Wednesday	Thursday	Friday	Saturday
Morning							
Lunch							
Dinner							

79

DISCLAIMER:

Please be advised that the information being presented here is based on other research with distressed dementia caregivers in the United States. We do not know if it will be equally effective with all families in the United States or families living in other parts of the world since to our knowledge, information pertaining to this question is not yet available. Further, we do not guarantee or promise that the techniques illustrated in this training workbook (and related website and DVD) will be helpful to every individual caregiver who follows this training. For example, the problems you are confronted with may be different from the ones presented here, or you may have so many problems that you are overwhelmed and in need of professional assistance in order to cope effectively with your situation.

This training workbook/website/DVD is not intended to substitute for medical judgment as to the cause of your problems. Furthermore, it is not intended to treat any medical or psychological problems you may have as a family caregiver. This training workbook/website/DVD is an educational tool only, to help you and your family learn more about Alzheimer's disease and to give you information about common ways to cope with associated problems.

Individuals with medical conditions should not use the "deep breathing" or any of the other techniques presented here for stress management without their doctor's advice and approval.

Not all of this information is suitable for everyone. To reduce the risk of injury, consult your doctor before beginning this or any caregiver program. The instructions and advice presented here are in no way intended as a substitute for family counseling, psychotherapy, or any form of medical treatment. The creators, producers, participants, and distributors of this program disclaim any liability or loss in connection with the exercise and advice herein.